MW01674737

Contents

Chapter 1

Preface

With all its exotic ingredients, unfamiliar dishes, and tongue-tingling flavors, Indian cuisine can be both exciting and intimidating. It's such a complete world of taste. You combine all the techniques from other cuisines and add magical spices to get a titillating food experience.

Indian cuisine uses the whole palette of flavors—spicy, sour, sweet, and hot all at the same time—making it something that wants to jump off the plate.

Don't be afraid to start playing around with cooking Indian food at home. First, it's important to understand the various dishes and flavors that make up Indian cuisine.

Chapter 2

Ingredients

2.1 Guide to Ingredients

Most of the ingredients are available at the grocery stores or supermarkets. Some, though, are special and have to be obtained from the Indian stores. Substitutes may change the character of the dish. It is better to omit an ingredient if not available than to substitute for it. If whole spice is not available, you may use the ground form, but the ground form is less pungent.

Name	Indian Name	Description
Asafoetida	Hing	Dried gum resin from the root of various Iranian and East Indian plants. Has a strong fetid odor—definitely an acquired taste. May be obtained.
Besan	Besan	Flour of dried chick peas.
Cardamom	Elaichi	Dried fruit of a plant. Mostly the seeds are used. Seeds of 4 pods measure approximately $\frac{1}{4}$ t.
Coriander	dhania	Aromatic herb of the parsley family. Sold as cilantro or chinese parsley. Also sold as seed or dry powder.
Cumin	Jeera	Very aromatic and reminiscent. Sold whole or ground.
Dals	Dal	Hindi name for all members of the legume or pulse family. Commonly used are: Arhar, Channa, Masur, Mung, Labia (black-eyed peas), Rajma (red kidney beans).

Fennel Seed	Sauf	Has an agreeable odor and licorice flavor. Available whole or ground.
Fenugreek	Methi	Has a pleasant bitter flavor and sweetish odor.
Garam Masala	Garam Masala	A mixture of spices; details come later.
Chat Masala	Chat Masala	A variation of Garam masala Available in Indian stores.
Ghee	Fat for frying.	Pure ghee is clarified butter.
Mustard oil	Larson	Pungent oil made from black mustard seeds.
Mint	Pudina	Aromatic herb. Fresh and dried leaves are used in the preparation of chutneys. Dried leaves are much less fragrant than the fresh ones.
Pomegranate	Anar dana	A flavoring agent. Has some scent.
Saffron	Kesar	Made of stigmas of a flower grown in Kashmir and Spain. It is aromatic and yields a yellow color.
Turmeric	Haldi	An aromatic powdered root. Used as a flavoring and for flavoring curries.

To make Garam Masala: (approximately 1 $\frac{1}{2}$ cups)

Quantity	**Ingredient**
3 - 5" pieces	Cinnamon stick
1 c (???)	Green cardamom pods
$\frac{1}{2}$ c	Cumin seed
$\frac{1}{2}$ c	Black pepper corns
$\frac{1}{2}$ c	Cloves
$\frac{1}{2}$ c	Coriander seeds

Procedure:
Dry the ingredients in an oven. Do not let them turn brown. Remove the seeds from the cardamom pods. Pound cinnamon sticks into smaller pieces. Combine ingredients until they are well mixed and blend at high speed for 2-3 minutes until completely pulverized (LINE MISSING, The recipe seems to be complete, but as the original had this I am letting it remain.)

Chapter 3

This and That

3.1 Onion and Tomato Raita

4-6 Servings

Quantity	Ingredient
8 oz.	Yogurt (plain)
1 small	Onion
$\frac{1}{2}$ t	Salt
1 small	Tomato
$\frac{1}{2}$ t	Chat Masala (optional)
$\frac{1}{2}$ t	Black pepper (ground)
$\frac{1}{4}$ c	Milk

1. Beat yogurt and milk until smooth.
2. Chop onion and tomatoes and add to yogurt.
3. Add salt and pepper and sprinkle the Chat Masala over, and serve.

3.2 Boondhi Raita

Quantity	Ingredient
$\frac{1}{4}$ c	Besan
$\frac{1}{2}$ c	Water
	Ghee for frying

to taste	Salt
to taste	Pepper
to taste	Chat Masala
$1\frac{1}{2}$ c	Yogurt
$\frac{1}{4}$ c	Milk

1. Make a pouring paste of the besan and water.
2. Heat ghee and drop paste into it through a slotted spoon to get little drops that fall one at a time (these are boondhi).
3. Remove the drops when golden brown and dry on a paper towel to remove extra oil.
4. Soak the drops in warm water.
5. Add milk, salt, pepper, and add Chat Masala to yogurt.
6. Squeeze water out of boondhi and add to yogurt.

3.3 Mint and Coriander Chutney

Quantity	**Ingredient**
1 bunch	Coriander leaves
1 bunch	Mint leaves
1	Green chili
1 oz.	Seedless tamarind
1 tsp	Salt
4 T	Water
1 medium	Onion

1. Wash and soak tamarind in water for $\frac{1}{2}$ hour.
2. Clean, pick and wash the coriander and mint.
3. Separate pulp from the tamarind and squeeze out the pulp.
4. Grind coriander, mint, green chili and onion into a fine paste.
5. Add the tamarind pulp and salt.

6. Blend well. In an airtight jar this can be refrigerated for up to one week.

Chapter 4

Breads

4.1 Chapati (Phulka)

for 4, serving 1 or 2

Quantity	Ingredient
1 c	Whole wheat flour (or $\frac{1}{3}$ white + $\frac{2}{3}$ whole wheat)
$\frac{1}{2}$ c	Water

1. Put flour in a large bowl with half the water.
2. Blend the two together until it holds.
3. Beat and knead well until it forms a compact ball.
4. Knead dough until it is smooth and elastic.
5. Set aside for 30 minutes.
6. Knead and divide dough into 4 to 6 parts.
7. Roll each ball into a tortilla like flat, about $\frac{1}{8}$" thick.
8. Heat an ungreased skillet.
9. Put phulka on it, and let it cook for about 1 minute (The top should just start to look dry and small bubbles should just start to form).
10. Turn and cook the second side for $\frac{2}{3}$ minutes until small bubbles form.

11. Turn again and cook the first side pressed lightly with a towel. It should puff. Serve warm (maybe slightly buttered).

Note: Since the rolled out chappati's will dry out if they are left to stand while cooking the others, it is advantageous to roll them out individually before cooking them.

4.2 Paratha

Quantity	**Ingredient**
1 c	Whole wheat flour
	Ghee
	Water

1. Make chappati dough.
2. Divide into 6 parts and make balls.
3. Flatten and roll each.
4. Spread ghee over them and fold.
5. Roll again.
6. Heat the paratha on a griddle like you would a chappati, but spread some ghee over the top side. Turn and spread ghee on the other side. Fry until the bottom is crisp and golden, then turn and fry the remaining side.
7. Repeat with all six.
8. Serve at once, since they lose crispness if stored.

4.3 Stuffed Parathas

Make dough for regular chappati's.

Fillings

1. **Potato -**
Boil potatoes, mash, add salt and chili to taste. Add Garam Masala and mango powder.

2. **Radish -**
   Grate one large Diakon Radish, add salt and leave for $\frac{1}{2}$ hour. Squeeze out all the water, add grated ginger, chili, and pomegranate seeds.

3. **Cauliflower -**
   Grate cauliflower, add salt, pepper, garlic, and Garam Masala.

Method

1. Roll out 2 small chappati's. Place filling on one, cover with the second, seal edges and cook as for parathas.

Chapter 5

Snacks

5.1 Bhel

This is a concoction that I often bought from street vendors in India. My mouth still waters whenever I think of Bhel. The recipe presented here was taken off the net, and I haven't had a chance to try it yet. I include the note from the contributors:

> *Warning: This recipe is directed at those who know what Bhelpuri tastes like, quantities mentioned are approximate, proportions are left to the reader's taste. Purists will have to go to an Indian grocery shop. Deviationists may use substitutes. The most important thing is to keep the puffed rice-sev mixture crisp by not adding the other ingredients to it until it is served. This should be done on the plate.*

Quantity	**Ingredient**
	Puffed Rice (1 carton of Rice Krispies may be used)
1 packet	Bhel mix or Sev
2 cups	Mashed boiled potatoes (mashed coarsely and then salted)
$\frac{1}{2}$ cup	Chopped fresh coriander leaves (a.k.a Chinese parsley)
3 Tbsp	Freshly roasted and ground cumin
to taste	Green chilies
1-2 Tbsp	Freshly ground black pepper
to taste	Tamarind
to taste	Jaggery (or Brown Sugar)
1 cup	Chopped onions.

Method

1. First boil the potatoes, mash them, salt them, and add pepper to taste. Add some coriander leaves too.
2. Roast the cumin and grind it.
3. Dissolve about 4 Tbsp of tamarind concentrate in 1 cup of hot water, and let it simmer and thicken gradually. Dissolve the jaggery (or sugar) until the sauce becomes tart and slightly sweet. (You may add some salt and ground red paprika, if you want to.) The sauce should be of a consistency slightly thinner than maple syrup. Pour into a serving container (like a creamer). Mix the puffed rice and sev/bhel mix in a large bowl.
4. On a plate, serve the rice-bhel mixture, add the potatoes, then the onions, chilies, and then dust the cumin powder over it. Next pour on the sauce and top with the coriander garnish. (Add salt/pepper to taste).
5. Mix the ingredients on the plate and eat.

5.2 Bonda With Instant Mashed Potato

This recipe was taken from Saranya Mandava's book on Indian cuisine.

Quantity	Ingredient
1 medium	Onion
2 cups	Potato buds
1 and $\frac{1}{2}$ cup	Peas and carrots
2 big ones	Green chilies
1 teaspoon	Lemon juice
1 cup	Gram flour
$\frac{1}{2}$ tea spoon	Mustard seed
pinch	Turmeric
$\frac{1}{2}$ teaspoon	Baking powder
$\frac{1}{4}$" piece	Ginger
1 small bunch	Coriander leaves
2 teaspoons	Salt

Oil

Method - The filling is prepared as follows:

1. Mix potato buds and $\frac{1}{2}$ teaspoon of salt with 1 cup of hot water.
2. Finely chop ginger, chilies, coriander leaves, and onion.
3. Heat oil (about 5 Tbsp) and add mustard seeds.
4. Add chopped ingredients and fry until onions are brown.
5. Add carrots, peas, turmeric and 1 tsp of salt and cook on low heat for about 10 minutes.
6. Add potato (now mashed) and fry for 5 minutes.
7. Remove from heat, add lemon juice and let cool.

Method - The batter is prepared as follows:

1. Combine gram flour, 3 Tbsp of oil, $\frac{3}{4}$ cup water, $\frac{1}{2}$ tsp salt, the baking powder and mix thoroughly
2. After the batter is prepared, make small balls out of the filling and roll them in the batter. Next fry it in hot oil. You will get about 20-30 small bondas.

5.3 Pakoras (Savory Fritters)

Quantity	Ingredient
Batter:	
$\frac{1}{2}$ c	Besan
5 oz.	Warm water
$\frac{1}{4}$ t	Red pepper
$\frac{3}{4}$ t	Salt
$\frac{1}{2}$ t	Garam Masala
	paprika (optional)
Vegetables:	
1	Small onion
1	Potato

	A few spinach leaves
	Oil for deep frying

Method

1. In a bowl put the besan and half the water, and stir until it becomes a thick batter. Beat hard for 5 minutes. gradually add the rest of the water, and leave to swell for 30 minutes. Add salt, pepper and Garam Masala and beat again.
2. Wash peel and slice the onion and potatoes.
3. Wash and pat dry the spinach leaves.
4. Heat oil until smoking hot, dip the vegetables in the batter and deep fry until golden brown.
5. Serve hot.

5.4 Dahi Vada (Savory Balls in Yogurt)

Quantity	Ingredient
$\frac{1}{2}$ c	Urad dal
$\frac{1}{2}$	Moong dal
1 c	Yogurt
	Spice to taste (cumin and paprika)
	Oil for frying
$\frac{1}{4}$ c	Milk

Method

1. Clean dal, wash and soak in water for 4 hours.
2. Blend in blender at medium speed using the minimum amount of water required to keep paste moving freely.
3. Add salt and start heating oil.
4. Drop spoonfuls of batter in the hot oil using a large tablespoon. Fry until golden brown.

5. Drop in water. Let it soak till ready to serve.

6. Beat yogurt with milk. Add spice according to taste. Squeeze out water from the vada and add yogurt. Serve.

5.5 Upma

Recipe from Sriram, 1985

This is a breakfast dish in the southern part of India. Ingredients

Quantity	**Ingredient**
1 cup	Cream of wheat
1	Onion cut lengthwise
1 teaspoon	Salt
$\frac{1}{4}$ teaspoon	Mustard seeds
$\frac{1}{8}$ teaspoon	Urad dal
1	Cashew-nut
$\frac{1}{4}$	Lemon
$\frac{1}{2}$ cup	Peas
1 clove	Garlic
1/10" piece	Ginger
1	Green chili cut into small pieces.

Method

1. Fry cream of wheat on a dry pan for 5 minutes and set aside.

2. Put two tablespoons of oil in a pan and heat.

3. Add mustard seeds, Urad dal, cashewnut, and garlic clove. Wait till mustard seeds stop splitting.

4. Add the onion, chili, and ginger and fry till the onion turns brown.

5. Add cream of wheat and fry for 3-5 minutes.

6. Add salt and peas.

7. Add two cups of boiling water and stir for 2 minutes. (Switch off the stove as soon as the water is poured.)

8. Cover the vessel for 4 minutes. Add lime if needed.

5.6 Vegetable Puff

12 puffs

This is a local Karnataka speciality.

Quantity	Ingredient
1	Ready to use pastry roll (Pepperidge farms)
	Mixed Vegetables. (potatoes, peas may be added)
to taste	Masala
	Green Chilies
to taste	Salt

Method

1. Cook a vegetable mix with potatoes, peas, green chilies and lots of Masala. Check for salt, before you stuff it in the pastry roll; no way to rectify it later.

2. Thaw the roll for about 10 minutes before unfolding.

3. After the pastry roll has thawed, open it out on a flat sheet and roll it with a pin to make it a little thinner. The pastry sheet would now be about 12" x 12".

4. Cut the sheet into 6 pieces.

5. Place about 2-3 Tbsp of the cooked vegetable onto the sheet and fold it around it. Seal all the corners, by pressing the sheets together and applying a little water.

6. Stick it into a pre-heated oven (350 $F°$) for about 20-30 minutes or until it browns. Make sure that you flip it around every 5-10 minutes.

Chapter 6

Vegetables

6.1 Gobi Aloo (Cauliflower and Potatoes)

This is my own recipe.

This recipe livens up ordinary cauliflower and potatoes into something quite different. The recipe shown here has spices that are not necessary (like cloves and cardamom) or at least that's not how mom made it at home, however it adds a nice touch.

Quantity	Ingredient
1	Large cauliflower
3	Medium sized potatoes
$\frac{1}{2}$ large	Onion sliced thinly in long slices
1 teaspoon	Mustard seeds
2 or 3 pods	Cardamom
1 teaspoon	Coriander
1 teaspoon	Cumin seeds
$\frac{1}{2}$ teaspoon	Turmeric
1	Bayleaf
3	Cloves
3 tablespoons	Vegetable Oil

Method

1. Start boiling the potatoes in a saucepan. Let them boil for at least 15 minutes. After they are done, turn off the heat and let them stand in the water.

2. Cut the cauliflower into small bite sized pieces (roughly 1" cubes), throwing away most of the stem pieces. Wash and drain in a collander.

3. While the potatoes are cooking, heat the oil in a wide skillet until it is very hot. Add the mustard seeds and wait until they start popping. Add bay leaves, cardamom and cloves.

4. Mix around for a while and then add onions. Wait until the onion starts to turn before adding the rest of the spices (except for turmeric).

5. Put the cauliflower in the skillet and fry in the oil and spices for 2 minutes. While the cauliflower is frying, cut up the potatoes into bite sized pieces and add to the skillet. Add turmeric and stir.

6. Continue stirring the vegetables under medium heat for another couple of minutes. Add $\frac{1}{2}$ cup of water and reduce heat to low. Cover skillet and let cook for 5 minutes.

7. Check tenderness of vegetables. If they are still too hard, add another $\frac{1}{4}$ cup of water and cover again for 5 minutes.

8. Salt to taste and serve.

6.2 Chole "Bill and Jim" (Chick Peas)

This recipe is named after Bill Chiles and Jim Muller both of whom liked my concoctions well enough that I started cooking this a lot. This is a real simple way of making chick peas. It barely takes 15 minutes and the result is quite delicious. Ask Jim and Bill.

Quantity	**Ingredient**
1 can	Chick peas (also called garbanzo beans) (Progresso is a good brand.)
1 large	Onion chopped finely
2 medium sized	Potatoes (optional)
1 teaspoon	Mustard seeds
2 or 3 pods	Cardamom
1 teaspoon	Coriander
1 teaspoon	Cumin seeds
1 tablespoon	Garam Masala

Vegetable Oil

Method

1. If you are using the potatoes, start boiling them in a saucepan. Let them boil for at least 15 minutes. After they are done, turn off the heat and let them stand in the water.
2. While the potatoes are cooking, heat the oil in a wide skillet until it is very hot. Add the mustard seeds and wait until they start popping. Add bay leaves, cardamom and cloves.
3. Mix around for a while and then add onions. Waituntill the onion starts to turn golden before adding the rest of the spices (except for the Garam Masala).
4. Add chick-peas with all the liquid. Cut up the potatoes into bite sized pieces and add to the skillet. Add Garam Masala.
5. Continue stirring the chick-peas under medium heat for 5-7 minutes without covering.
6. Check the tenderness of the potatoes. If they are still too hard, add another $\frac{1}{4}$ cup of water and cook for another couple of minutes.
7. Salt to taste and serve.

6.3 Masaledar Sem (Spicy Green Beans)

Serves 6

This recipe is mostly Madhur Jaffrey's, although I don't follow it to the letter when I cook anymore. I like to serve the beans a little crunchier than you would find in an indian home, so I don't cook it as much in the end. It definitely warrants experimentation. This recipe is guaranteed to spice up an ordinary meal. It also goes well with plain rice and meat or chicken that has been prepared simply.

Quantity	Ingredient
1 $\frac{1}{2}$ lb.	Green beans (Trim the ends and then cut the beans in half crosswise.)

$1\frac{1}{2}$" long and 1" thick piece	Fresh ginger (Peel and chop coarsely.)
10 cloves	Garlic peeled
1 cup	Water
4 tablespoons	Vegetable oil
3 teaspoons	Whole cumin seeds
2 teaspoons	Ground coriander seeds
2 medium	Tomatoes, peeled (put tomatoes in very hot water for a few seconds, peel off the skin and finely chop.)
to taste	Salt
	Freshly ground pepper
3 tablespoons	Lemon juice (or to taste)

Method

1. Put ginger and garlic into a food processor and add $\frac{1}{2}$ cup water. Blend until fairly smooth.

2. Heat the oil in a wide, heavy saucepan over a medium flame. When hot, put in the cumin seeds. Stir for half a minute.

3. Pour in the ginger-garlic paste. Stir and cook for about two minutes. Put in the coriander and stir a few times.

4. Put in the chopped tomatoes. Stir and cook for 2 minutes while mashing the tomato pieces with the back of a slotted spoon.

5. Put in the beans and salt and one cup of water and simmer them.

6. Cover, turn heat to low and cook for 8-10 minutes or until the beans are tender.

7. Remove the cover. Add the lemon juice and a generous amount of freshly ground pepper.

8. Turn up the heat and boil away the remaining liquid, stirring the beans gently as you do so.

6.4 Vegetable Kurma

This Recipe from Sriram

Quantity	**Ingredient**
2 cups	Vegetables
2	Onions cut length-wise
2	Green chilies cut length-wise
1 teaspoon	Coriander powder
1 and $\frac{1}{4}$ teaspoon	Salt
one pinch	Turmeric powder
$\frac{1}{2}$"	Cinnamon stick
2	Cloves
2	Cardamom
2 tablespoons	Coconut powder
1 teaspoon	Khus-Khus (poppy seeds)
$\frac{1}{4}$ teaspoon (3 cloves)	Garlic
$\frac{1}{4}$ teaspoon powder (or $\frac{1}{2}$" fresh)	Ginger

Method

1. Put a reasonable sized vessel on the range and heat oil.
2. Add cinnamon, cloves and cardamom and fry for 2-3 minutes.
3. Add onions and green chilies and fry till onions turn brown.
4. Add garlic + ginger paste and fry for a minute or so.
5. Add vegetables and fry for about 3 minutes.
6. Add Water (about a cup or two).
7. Let the vegetables + turmeric powder cook.
8. If you are using canned or frozen vegetables skip the above step.
9. Add coconut paste, khus-khus, salt and wait until cooked. (note: Cook on low heat.)

6.5 Vegetable Curry

Recipe from Sriram, 1985

Quantity	**Ingredient**
1 cup	Vegetables
$\frac{1}{4}$-$\frac{1}{2}$ teaspoon	Coriander powder
$\frac{1}{8}$-$\frac{1}{4}$ teaspoon	Chili powder
$\frac{1}{8}$-$\frac{1}{4}$ teaspoon	Garlic powder
1 teaspoon	Salt
1	large Onion
$\frac{1}{4}$-$\frac{1}{2}$ teaspoon	Mustard seeds
$\frac{1}{8}$ teaspoon	Urad Dal
$\frac{1}{4}$-$\frac{1}{2}$ cup	Tomatoes-crushed

Method

1. Mix the garlic, coriander and the chili powder along with salt and place it aside.
2. Pour about 2 tablespoons of oil in a pan and heat.
3. Add mustard seeds and urad dal. The mustard seeds will split and the oil may spill. Be careful when you are doing this. Wait until the mustard seeds stop making any noise.
4. Add onions and fry until the onions turn brown.
5. Add the vegetables, the mixture of step 1 and the crushed tomatoes.
6. Fry for about 5 minutes, if you are using canned vegetables. Otherwise cover the pan and let the vegetables cook. (This might take about 10-15 min.)

6.6 Green Pepper Curry

This recipe from Sriram

Quantity	Ingredient
2 large ones	Green Pepper
$\frac{1}{4}$ teaspoon	Chili powder
$\frac{1}{8}$ teaspoon	Turmeric powder
$\frac{1}{2}$ teaspoon	Dhania powder
1 tablespoon	Coconut flakes
1 teaspoon	Khus Khus (poppy seeds)
1 small bunch	Fresh Coriander leaves
2 small	Tomatoes
2	Onions
2 tablespoons	Oil
1 small piece	Vadium[a]
1 $\frac{1}{4}$ teaspoon	Salt

[a]Vadium is a combination of various spices.

Method

1. Cut the green peppers, onion and tomatoes lengthwise.
2. Grind chili-powder, turmeric, dhania powder, coconut and poppy seeds.
3. Heat oil and add vadium.
4. When vadium turns brown, add onions and fry for 4 minutes.
5. Add tomatoes and fry for 2 minutes.
6. Add green pepper and Masala.
7. Add coriander leaves.
8. Cook on low heat (should take around 15 minutes).

6.7 Dry Potatoes (Sookha Aloo)

4-6 Servings

Quantity	Ingredient
4 medium size	Potatoes
2 t	Cumin seeds

1 t	Salt
2 t	Mango powder
$\frac{1}{4}$ t	Hot pepper
2 t	Garam Masala
	Oil (to fill pan to 2")

Method

1. Boil potatoes until cooked but not overdone.
2. Peel and cut into $\frac{1}{2}$" cubes.
3. Heat oil very hot, add and brown cumin seeds.
4. Add potatoes and fry until they are golden brown. Add the remaining ingredients, and fry for 2-3 minutes or more. Remove from oil with a slotted spoon.
5. Serve hot.

Tips: Use enough oil so that the potatoes will not need to be stirred often. This avoids breaking them up.

6.8 Okra (Bhindi)

Serves 6

Quantity	Ingredient
1 lb	okra
2 small	Onions
2 small	Tomatoes
$\frac{1}{4}$ t	Turmeric
to taste	Salt
	Red pepper (optional)
	Oil for frying

Method

1. Wash the okra and dry it thoroughly.

2. Cut off the heads and cut into small circles.

3. Chop the onions and tomatoes separately.

4. Deep fry the okra until very brown.

5. Remove from heat and set aside. Pour out some oil.

6. Add turmeric to hot oil. Add the onions and fry until golden brown.

7. Add the fried okra, salt, pepper, and tomatoes.

8. Cover and bake at 250 $F°$ for 15 minutes.

6.9 Paneer (Cheese)

Quantity	**Ingredient**
1 $\frac{1}{2}$ pints	Milk
$\frac{1}{2}$ t	White vinegar **AND**
$\frac{1}{2}$ t	Lemon juice **OR**
1 c	Yogurt

Method

1. Heat milk and stir constantly to prevent a layer of cream from forming on the top.

2. Remove from heat when it boils and slowly add white vinegar and lemon juice or yogurt. This sours the milk.

3. Strain through a muslin cloth or a double layer of cheese cloth and squeeze out the whey (liquid).

4. Hang to drip dry for 2-3 hours (or overnight). Then lay out the cheese in a rectangle in a tray and place a weight (the more the better, but at least 10 lbs) on it for $\frac{3}{4}$ hour.

5. Cut it into whatever shape you like.

6.10 Mattar Paneer (Peas & Cheese)

Quantity	Ingredient
2	Onions
2	Tomatoes
4 cloves	Garlic
$\frac{1}{2}$ packet frozen	Peas
1" cube	Ginger
$\frac{1}{4}$ t	Turmeric
to taste	Salt
to taste	Pepper
$\frac{1}{2}$ t	Garam Masala
2 c	Water

Method

1. Cut paneer in 1" cubes and deep fry.
2. Make Masala with onion, garlic, ginger, and tomatoes.
3. Season and add turmeric.
4. Add peas and paneer.

6.11 Navrathna Kurma

Serves 6

Quantity	Ingredient
100 grams	Paneer (or cottage cheese)
2 teacups	Mixed boiled vegetables (carrots, french beans, green peas, potatoes)
3	Tomatoes
2	Onions
1 t	Ginger and garlic paste
$1\frac{1}{2}$ t	Chili powder
$\frac{1}{2}$ t	Turmeric powder
2 t	Coriander powder
1 t	Garam Masala
1 teacup	Milk

3 t	Fresh cream
3 t	Ghee
to taste	Salt
	Ghee for deep frying

Method

1. Grate the onions.
2. Put the tomatoes in hot water. After 10 minutes take off the skin and chop.
3. Cut the paneer into small pieces and deep fry in ghee.
4. Heat oil in a vessel and fry the onions for a few minutes.
5. Add the ginger and garlic paste, and fry for $\frac{1}{2}$ minute.
6. Add the chopped tomatoes, turmeric powder, coriander powder and chili powder, Garam Masala and salt. Fry for at least 3-4 minutes.
7. Add the boiled vegetables, milk, cream and fried paneer pieces.
8. Cook for a few minutes.
9. Serve hot decorated with silver foil.

6.12 Cauliflower and Potatoes (Aloo Gobi)

Quantity	Ingredient
1 medium	Cauliflower
2 medium	Potatoes
1	Onion
1	Tomato
1 clove	Garlic
1" piece	Ginger
pinch	Turmeric
to taste	Salt
to taste	Pepper
to taste	Garam Masala

Method

1. Make Masala with onion, garlic, ginger, and tomatoes.
2. Add turmeric and spices.
3. Break the cauliflower in flowerettes and cut the potatoes into cubes (8 pieces each).
4. Add both to Masala and lower heat to simmer. Cover the pot until the cauliflower and potatoes are coated.

6.13 Curried eggplant (Bhartha)

Serves 4 to 6

Quantity	Ingredient
2 lb.	Eggplant
4 medium	Tomatoes
3 t	Fresh chopped coriander
$\frac{1}{2}$ c	Ghee
$\frac{1}{2}$ c	Finely chopped onion

Method

1. Preheat oven to 450 F°.
2. Bake in the middle level of the oven for 1 hour or until very tender.
3. While they are still warm, peel and crush the eggplants.
4. Heat oil and fry onions until soft and clear. Do not brown.
5. Add the tomatoes and fry for 2 minutes.
6. Add the eggplant and stir until almost all liquid disappears and the mixture leaves the side.
7. place into a bowl, sprinkle on coriander and serve at once.

6.14 Curried Mushrooms

Quantity	**Ingredient**
$\frac{1}{2}$ lb.	Mushrooms
1 large	Onion
$\frac{1}{4}$ t	Turmeric
to taste	Salt
to taste	Chili
2 large	Tomatoes
	Oil

Method

1. Wash and finely slice mushrooms. Slice onion fine.
2. Heat oil and add turmeric and onions. Fry until soft.
3. Add the sliced tomatoes and cook for 3 minutes, stirring all the time.
4. Add the mushrooms, cover and simmer for 15-20 minutes.
5. Remove cover and dry out all the water.
6. Serve hot.

Chapter 7

Lentils

This chapter needs more recipes about Dals. For now, I only have a recipe for 'sambar' a thin dal recipe from South India. This is typically served with idlis or plain rice. Idlis are hard to make and I haven't been able to find a satisfactory recipe for them to date.

7.1 Sambhar

This recipe from Sriram

Quantity	**Ingredient**
1 cup	Toor Dal
1 teaspoon	Tamarind
3 teaspoons	Salt
a pinch	Turmeric
2 teaspoons	Channa Dal
3 teaspoons	Dhania seeds
1 pinch	Hing
3	Red chilies
$\frac{1}{4}$ cup	Grated coconut
1 teaspoon	Mustard
10	Coriander leaves
1	Green peppers cut into pieces
1	Onion chopped
1	Tomato cut into pieces

Method

1. Boil the toor dal with 3 cups of water.
2. Fry channa dal, dhania seeds, hing, and red chilies for a few minutes, and then fry them with the grated coconut.
3. Grind the above mixture with water.
4. Fry the green pepper in oil for a few minutes.
5. Boil the tamarind paste, water, salt, turmeric, tomato and vegetables.
6. Add ??? 3 ??? and cook for about 5 minutes.
7. Add boiled dal and bring it to a boil
8. In the meantime fry the mustard seeds and onion.
9. Add the above ingredients & coriander leaves to the mixture.

7.2 Masur Dal (Lentils)

Serves 4

Quantity	Ingredient
1 c	Dal (Moong - yellow, or masur - pink)
3 $\frac{1}{2}$ c	Water
to taste	Salt
to taste	Pepper
$\frac{1}{4}$ teaspoon	Turmeric
2 cloves	Garlic
1" piece	Ginger
1 small	Onion
2-3 Tablespoons	Ghee (Can be replaced by butter)
1 t	Cumin seed

Method

1. Wash the dal and drain it.

2. Boil water and add the dal, salt, pepper, turmeric, finely chopped ginger, and garlic. Cover the pot and simmer for 20 minutes.

3. When done, heat the ghee, add the cumin and fry until golden brown. Add thinly sliced onions. Fry until crisp and brown.

You may add paprika and finely chopped tomatoes to the above for color (Pour over the dal and serve).

7.3 Mah Ki Dal (Whole Black Beans)

Quantity	**Ingredient**
1 c	Urad or Mah dal
1" piece	Ginger
12 cloves	Garlic
	Water
to taste	Salt
2-3 Tablespoons	Ghee (Can be replaced by butter)
to taste	Green chili (optional)
to taste	Garam Masala
*frac*14 t	Turmeric

Method

1. Clean, wash and add the dal to boiling water.

2. Add turmeric, salt, half of the finely chopped ginger, garlic and cook on medium heat for 2-3 hours or pressure cook at 15psi for $\frac{1}{2}$ hour.

3. Uncover, cook further in same pan on low heat for $\frac{1}{2}$ hour, stir and mash every now and then until a creamy consistency is achieved.

4. Heat the ghee, add remaining ginger, stir, add sliced onions, chili, and fry until golden brown.

5. Add cumin or coriander (optional). Pour over dal just before serving.

7.4 Red Kidney Beans (Rajma)

Serves 6 - 8

Quantity	Ingredient
2 c	Red kidney beans
3 qt.	Water
1 t	Turmeric
1 T	Salt
$\frac{1}{4}$ c	Oil
1 c	Onion, Chopped
1" piece	Ginger, chopped
1 t	Garam Masala
3	Chopped tomatoes
	Coriander leaves for garnish

Method

1. Wash beans and boil for 2-3 hours or $\frac{1}{2}$ hour in a pressure cooker.
2. In the meantime make Masala of onions, garlic, ginger and tomato as in chicken curry.
3. Add to the beans and cook again until most of the liquid dries up and the beans are soft and thoroughly cooked.
4. Garnish with coriander leaves and serve.

7.5 Curried Garbanzo Beans

Quantity	Ingredient
8 oz.	Garbanzo beans
to taste	Green chili (optional)
12 cloves	Garlic
2" piece	Ginger
to taste	Pepper
1 large	Cardamom
6	Cloves
1"	Cinnamon stick

to taste	Salt
	Paprika
4 oz.	Oil
	Mango powder
3	Onions
	Dried pomegranate seeds
4	Tomatoes

Method

1. Clean, wash and soak the beans overnight.
2. Boil them in the same water with salt, 1 small finely chopped onion, 4 cloves garlic, 4 large cardamom, a 1" piece of ginger and 6 cloves.
3. Simmer in pan about an hour or until tender, or pressure cook for 7 minutes at 15 psi.
4. Heat oil. Fry thinly sliced remaining onions and cloves of garlic. Cook until mixture browns and dries up. Add finely chopped tomatoes and cook 4-5 minutes more.
5. Add the beans and cook for 10 minutes more. Add the mango powder and pomegranate seeds, grated ginger and simmer over low heat for 15-20 minutes.
6. Before serving, pour 1 oz. (2 T) sizzling ghee over the beans.

Chapter 8

Rice

8.1 Chicken Pullao

Recipe from Sriram, 1985

Quantity	**Ingredient**
2 large	Onions cut lengthwise
2 large	Chilies cut lengthwise
2 c	Basmathi rice (about $\frac{1}{2}$ kg. (1 kilogram=2.2lbs)
1 large	Tomato (cut into small pieces)
10-15	Coriander leaves
5	Mint leaves
1 clove	Garlic
1" piece	Ginger
$\frac{1}{2}$ cup	Coconut powder
3 teaspoons	Salt
3-4	Cloves
2	Cardamom
1	Bay leaf
1"	Cinnamon stick
1 c	Yogurt
2 tablespoons	Butter
1 lb.	Boneless chicken

Method

1. Heat vessel with butter.

2. Fry bay leaves, cloves, cardamom and cinnamon.
3. Put onions and chilies in vessel and fry on low heat until onions turn brown.
4. Add ginger + garlic paste and fry until oil separates.
5. Add tomato and fry for 1 minute.
6. Add chicken + salt + yogurt and fry for one minute.
7. Add mint + coriander leaves.
8. Cover and cook until the gravy becomes semi-solid.
9. Cook rice in a separate vessel.
10. Put rice into chicken and mix (It is advisable to cook rice about $\frac{3}{4}$ths and then let it cook with the chicken).
11. Remove and serve (Will serve about 4 hungry grad. students.)

8.2 South Indian Pullav (Rice)

From Sriram, 1985

Quantity	Ingredient
1 c	Rice (Preferably Basmathi rice)
$\frac{1}{3}$ c	Tomato puree
1 large	Onion
1 c	Vegetables (preferably peas and carrots)
$\frac{1}{4}$-$\frac{1}{2}$ teaspoon	Coriander powder (also called dhania powder)
$\frac{1}{8}$-$\frac{1}{4}$ teaspoon	Garlic powder or
1 and a half cloves garlic	
$\frac{1}{8}$-$\frac{1}{4}$ teaspoon	Ginger powder
$\frac{1}{4}$" piece	Ginger
$\frac{1}{8}$-$\frac{1}{4}$ teaspoon	Chili powder
1	Green chili cut into small pieces
1-2 pieces	Cardamom
1 piece	Cloves
$\frac{1}{4}$" stick or $\frac{1}{8}$ teaspoon powder	Cinnamon

1	Bay leaf
1 teaspoon	Salt
1 teaspoon	Coriander leaves (if needed)

Method

1. Clean the rice with water and set aside.

2. Cut the onions length wise.

3. Fry the onions and cardamom in butter for about 4 minutes. If you are using green chili, then add the chili.

4. Add bay leaf, cloves, cinnamon and fry until the onions turn golden brown (This will probably take another 4-5 minutes).

5. Add the garlic and ginger paste (preferably prepared from fresh ginger and garlic).

6. Add dhania powder and chili powder (if green chili was not added before).

7. Add the tomato paste and one cup of water (you have to experiment with the quantity of water needed. I found 1-$\frac{1}{2}$ cups to be optimal) and bring the mixture to boil.

8. Add the vegetables, rice and salt.

9. If you like coconut, add $\frac{1}{4}$ cup of coconut flakes.

10. Reduce the flame and cover the vessel.

11. After about 4 minutes, stir the mixture.

12. Cover the lid again and wait until cooked (might take about 10-15 minutes).

13. Sprinkle on the coriander leaves in the end.

8.3 Vegetable Pullav 2

Recipe from Sriram, 1985 This recipe is slightly spicer than the previous one.

Quantity	Ingredient
1 c	Rice
1 $\frac{1}{2}$ c	Water
1 c	Vegetables
$\frac{1}{2}$"	Cinnamon stick
2	Cloves
2	Cardamom
1 $\frac{1}{4}$ teaspoon	Salt
$\frac{1}{8}$ teaspoon	Turmeric powder
1 teaspoon	Dhania powder
2	Chilies or
$\frac{1}{4}$ teaspoon powder	
$\frac{1}{2}$ can or 1 lb. (16 oz)	Tomatoes
$\frac{1}{2}$ cup	Coconut
1 bunch	Coriander leaves
4 cloves	Garlic
$\frac{1}{2}$" piece	Ginger (made into a paste)
2 tablespoons	Butter
1	Onion cut lengthwise

Method

1. Wash the rice and drain the water.
2. Extract one cup of water from tomatoes.
3. Pour the butter into a vessel and heat.
4. Add cinnamon, cardamom and cloves.
5. Add onions and chilies and fry until onions turn golden brown.
6. Add ginger + garlic paste and turmeric powder paste and fry until you get a nice smell.
7. Now pour in the tomato water + 1 cup water.

8. Add coconut, coriander powder (Dhania powder), salt and let boil
9. Add rice + coriander leaves + vegetables.
10. Reduce to low heat and let the rice cook.

8.4 Saffron Rice (Kesar Chawal)

Quantity	Ingredient
2 c	Rice
4 c	Water
6 T	Ghee
1 t	Saffron threads (or less)
2 T	Hot water
1 c	Sliced onion
1 small	Cinnamon stick - splintered
4	Bay leaves
4 large	Black cardamoms
1 T	Cumin seed
4	Cloves
2 t	Salt

Method

1. Soak saffron in hot water.
2. Wash and soak rice in 3 c water (optional).
3. Heat ghee and fry onions and then remove and keep aside.
4. Add cinnamon, cumin seeds, cardamoms, cloves and salt. Wait 1 minute and then add the bay leaves and $\frac{1}{2}$ the onions. Drain the rice and reserve the water.
5. Add the rice grains and stir for 4-5 minutes until all the water evaporates and the grains of rice are coated with oil.
6. Add the water and bring to a boil.
7. Add saffron and its water and pressure cook at 15 psi.
8. Remove from the heat and allow the pressure to drop by itself.

8.5 Navrattan Pullao (Nine-Jeweled Rice)

Quantity	Ingredient
1 c	Basmathi rice
1 $\frac{3}{4}$ c	Water
$\frac{1}{4}$ c	Oil
1 small	Finely sliced onion
6	Cloves
1"	Cinnamon stick
1 t	Salt
$\frac{1}{2}$ t	Cumin seed

For Mixing with rice before serving:

A $\frac{1}{4}$ c frozen peas (boiled), salt, 6 drops green food coloring mixed with 1 t water.

B $\frac{1}{4}$ c diced tomatoes, $\frac{1}{4}$ t red pepper, salt, Garam Masala, 6 drops red food coloring mixed in 2 t water.

Quantity	Ingredient
1	Thinly sliced onion
2 $\frac{1}{4}$ c	Ghee
1 oz.	Almonds
1 oz.	Cashew nuts
1 $\frac{1}{2}$ oz.	Golden raisins
1 oz.	Pistachio nuts
1" piece	Ginger thinly sliced
1	Green chili (optional)
1	Hard boiled egg

Method

1. Clean, wash, and soak rice in 1 $\frac{3}{4}$ c water for pressure cooking, or in 2 cups of water for pan cooking.

2. Heat oil and fry the onions. Add whole spices. Fry 1 minute. Add rice and fry for $\frac{2}{3}$ minutes to coat the rice grains with oil. Add the water which the rice was soaking in. Pressure cook, building up the pressure to 15 psi and let drop, OR cook in a pan bringing to full boil then down to a simmer followed by 20 minutes of cooking until the rice is done.

3. Divide rice into three parts. Thoroughly mix A with one part and B with another. Leave the last part plain. Keep rice separate and warm in the oven.

4. (C) Meanwhile fry the onion until it is crisp. Remove and fry almonds, cashew nuts, pistachios, raisins, ginger and chili. Chop egg and sprinkle with salt. Keep warm until required.

5. To serve, place onions, nuts, chopped egg and all of (C) in a dish and spread the three batches of rice in clumps above it aesthetically.

Chapter 9

Fish

9.1 Prawn (Shrimp) Curry

This Recipe from Sriram, 1985

Quantity	Ingredient
$\frac{1}{2}$ kg=1.1 lb.	Prawns
2	Onions diced into small pieces
$\frac{1}{4}$"	Cinnamon stick
$\frac{1}{4}$ teaspoon	Chili powder
$\frac{1}{2}$ teaspoon	Dhania powder
$\frac{1}{4}$ teaspoon	Garlic powder
$\frac{1}{2}$ teaspoon	ginger powder
1 bunch	Fresh coriander
1 teaspoon	Salt
$\frac{1}{4}$ teaspoon	Turmeric powder
1 tablespoon	Oil

Method

1. Clean the prawns and squeeze out the water.
2. Add chili, dhania, garlic, ginger, turmeric powder, salt and mix well.
3. Boil prawns on low heat.
4. Add 1 teaspoon of oil to the boiling prawns.

5. When water evaporates and the prawns are dry remove from the stove.
6. Heat the oil and put in the cinnamon.
7. Add prawns and fry for 2 minutes.
8. Add onions and fry until they turn brown.
9. Sprinkle on coriander leaves, remove from the heat and serve.

9.2 Coriander Fish (Bharia Machli)

Quantity	**Ingredient**
4 lb.	Sole, flounder, rock cod, or any other white whole fish
8 cloves	Garlic
3	Hot chilies (optional) (or cayenne)
1" piece	Ginger
1 medium bunch	Coriander
1 T	Coriander seeds
1 t	Brown sugar
1 t	Turmeric
$\frac{1}{2}$ t	Black mustard
$\frac{1}{2}$ t	Fenugreek seeds
1 T	Salt
$\frac{1}{2}$ c	Lemon juice
$\frac{1}{2}$ c	Vegetable oil
2 c	Chopped onion
1 c	Chopped tomato
$\frac{1}{2}$ t	Garam Masala

Method

1. Preheat oven to 400 F°.
2. Wash and pat fish dry. Sprinkle 1 t salt inside and set aside.
3. Blend garlic, chili, ginger, $\frac{1}{2}$ the coriander, coriander seeds, brown sugar, turmeric, mustard seeds, fenugreek seeds, salt and lemon juice until it all becomes a smooth paste (Add some water if needed).
4. Fry onions until they are soft and golden brown.

5. Add the blended Masala and cook until most of the liquid is gone, and it starts to leave the sides of the pan.

6. Add the tomatoes and Garam Masala. Fry for 2 minutes more and remove.

7. Coat one side of fish, stuff 1 $\frac{1}{2}$ cups inside. Close opening, spread the rest of the Masala over it. Cover tightly and bake for about 25 minutes.

8. Grill for 1-2 minutes in the broiler, and sprinkle on the remaining coriander.

9. Serve.

Chapter 10

Chicken

10.1 Mughlai Chicken with Almonds

This recipe is taken from Madhur Jaffrey's book

Quantity	Ingredient
1" piece	Ginger
8 to 9 cloves	Garlic
6 tablespoons	Blanched Almonds
7 tablespoons	Vegetable oil
1"	Cinnamon stick
2	Bay leaves
5	Cloves
10 pods	Cardamom
2 medium	Onions (cut into small pieces)
2 teaspoons	Ground cumin seeds
$\frac{1}{8}$-$\frac{1}{2}$ teaspoon	Red pepper
7 tablespoons	Yogurt
1 small carton	Whipped Cream
$\frac{1}{4}$ teaspoon	Garam Masala
2-2$\frac{1}{2}$ lbs.	Chicken boneless (2 trays of holy farms)
2 $\frac{1}{2}$ teaspoons	Salt
one bunch	Coriander leaves

Method

1. Grind the ginger, garlic, and almonds with water.

2. Heat oil in a non-stick pan, and fry the chicken until it turns golden brown. Keep it aside and drain the oil.
3. Heat some oil and add the cardamom, bay leaves and cloves and fry until the bay leaves turn brown.
4. Add the onions and fry for a few minutes.
5. Pour the paste from the blender and fry for a couple of minutes until the oil separates.
6. Add 1 tablespoon of yogurt and fry for 30 seconds. Keep adding tablespoons of yogurt and fry until you get a consistent mixture.
7. Add the chicken, whipped cream and salt and cook gently (low heat) for 20 minutes.
8. Add Garam Masala and coriander leaves and cook for another 10 minutes.

10.2 Malai Chicken

Recipe from Sriram, 1985

Quantity	**Ingredient**
1	Tray chicken
1	Chopped onion
1 small can	Tomato paste
1	Red Chili
2	Cloves
2	Cardamom
$\frac{1}{2}$"	Cinnamon stick
1	Bay leaf
1 carton	Light whipping cream
1 tsp	Dhania powder
$\frac{1}{2}$ tsp	Cumin powder
1 tsp	Garam Masala
1-1 $\frac{1}{4}$ tsp	Chili powder
$\frac{1}{2}$" piece	Ginger made into a paste
6 cloves	Garlic (made into paste)
	Fresh coriander

to taste	Salt
	Turmeric

Method

1. Heat oil.
2. Add red chili, cloves, cardamom, cinnamon stick, and bay leaf, and cook until the bay leaf turns golden brown.
3. Add the onion and fry for two minutes.
4. Add the ginger garlic paste and fry for 4 - 6 minute.
5. Add the chicken and fry for 5 minutes.
6. Sprinkle in chili, dhania powder, cumin powder and turmeric.
7. Cover chicken + salt (add water if needed) and cook for around 15 minutes until $\frac{3}{4}$ cooked.
8. Add can of tomato paste and cook on low heat.
9. Just before removing, add the whipping cream and cook for a few minutes.
10. Add Garam Masala and coriander leaves
11. Remove after a couple of minutes.

10.3 Chicken Curry North Indian Style

My own, mostly from mom's but synthesized with recipes from other friends.

Quantity	**Ingredient**
1 lb.	Chicken-drumsticks, thighs, breast pieces
1 small carton	Plain yogurt
2 medium	Onions very finely chopped
4 tbl	Vegetable oil
2	Cloves
$\frac{1}{2}$ tsp	Mustard powder
2 pods	Cardamom

$\frac{1}{2}$ tsp	Cumin powder
1 tsp	Garam Masala
1 tsp	Chili Powder
$\frac{1}{2}$" piece	Ginger
4 cloves	Garlic
$\frac{1}{3}$ tsp	Coriander Seeds
to taste	Salt
$\frac{1}{2}$ tsp	Freshly ground pepper

Method

1. Remove fat from the chicken and then salt and pepper it. Sprinkle with chili powder. Add yogurt and mix well until the chicken is covered liberally with yogurt. Use your hands. Set aside for 1 hour before cooking. If kept in the refrigerator, set aside for at least 4 hours.

2. Heat oil in a large heavy pan. When oil is hot, add mustard seeds, if you are using them. Add cloves, cardamom, and coriander seeds and fry for 30 seconds.

3. Add the onion and fry for two minutes until the onion beings to turn brown. Lower heat to medium.

4. Add the ginger and garlic paste and fry for 4-6 minutes.

5. Add mustard powder, if using it, add Garam Masala, and add cumin powder.

6. Brush excess yogurt off the chicken and put it in a large pot. Add ingredients from the frying pan. Cook uncovered over high heat for 4 minutes.

7. Reduce heat to low and cover. Cook for 25 minutes or until the chicken is tender, stirring every 5 minutes.

Important note: When chicken is cooked with a cover on the pot, it releases water that becomes a part of the sauce. If after 10 minutes, there isn't enough sauce in the pot, add $\frac{1}{4}$ cup water. Conversely, if there is too much liquid in the pot, cook uncovered until the liquid evaporates.

Variations: There are several variations to the above recipe:

1. Leave out the yogurt. Add $\frac{1}{4}$ cup of water just before turning the heat to low and covering the pot.

2. Boil two potatoes for 10 minutes before slicing them thinly. Add sliced potatoes to the pot when you start cooking the chicken.

3. This variation is usually called "Malai Chicken" or literally "creamy" chicken. Leave out the yogurt. When the chicken is $\frac{3}{4}$ done, add one small can of tomato paste. Just before removing add a small carton of whipping cream, and cook for a few minutes.

10.4 Chicken Curry (Murga)

4-6 Servings

Quantity	Ingredient
2-2 $\frac{1}{2}$ lb.	Skinned chicken
1 t	Garam Masala
3 t	Salt
1 c	Finely chopped tomato
$\frac{1}{4}$ c	Vegetable oil
$\frac{1}{2}$ c	Water
1 $\frac{1}{2}$ c	Finely chopped onion
1 $\frac{1}{2}$ t	Fresh ginger, chopped
1 t	Finely chopped garlic
1 t	Vinegar
1	Dried chili (optional)

Method

1. Cut chicken, separate legs and thighs, back and split breast.

2. Heat oil over high heat. Add onions and fry until golden brown. Take care not to burn them.

3. Add garlic, ginger and tomatoes. Fry until a smooth paste is obtained.

4. Add chicken, add water, bring to a boil, and add salt. Cover pot and lower heat. Add chili to make it hot if desired.

5. Stir constantly to avoid burning and coat the chicken pieces evenly.

6. After the chicken is done, add vinegar and cook for another 5 minutes on very low heat. Sprinkle on Garam Masala and serve.

10.5 Tandoori Chicken

2-3 Servings

Quantity	Ingredient
6 pieces	Thawed chicken, skinned
2 tsp	Ground Coriander
2 tsp	Masala (Tandoori paste is available)
to taste	Red pepper powder
Dash	Garlic powder
to taste	Salt
1 tsp	Ground jeera
	Soy sauce (or yogurt) (needed only if tandoori masala is used)

Method

1. If you are using the ready made tandoori paste then life is a lot easier. Replace all occurences of masala and soy sauce(or yogurt) with the tandoori paste.

2. Take the chicken and make *deep* cuts in it (so that the Masalas seeps in quickly).

3. If you are using soy sauce as the base, put some on the chicken pieces and let it seep in the cuts.

4. Rub in the Masalas as a mixture or one at a time. The idea is to let the Masalas seep in the cuts with the soy sauce. You can leave it for little while to seep in.

5. If you are using yogurt, you'll get a more authentic taste since the original TC is after all marinated in it. In this case, mix the Masalas in the yogurt first and then rub the stuff into the chicken cuts as before. The yogurt tends to leave a considerable amount of water behind. DON'T THROW THIS AWAY. Let it evaporate in the oven

with the chicken. This will keep the pieces from getting dry if overcooked. I have not faced the same problem with the soy sauce version (of dry chicken).

6. Cook the chicken until it starts turning brown. and the cuts you made start "expanding."

Notes: You may use any other interesting sauce as the base. Some previous experiences of my own are: Teriyaki (my Japaani-tandoori), Oriental sauce (my supermarket-tandoori).

Chapter 11

Lamb and Beef

11.1 Lamb Vindaloo

From Esquire Magazine, 1986: I have made the recipe a couple of times and both times with very good results. The finished dish is a spicy lamb dish that is quite exquisite. Be warned that this recipe takes quite a bit of effort to put together.

Quantity	**Ingredient**
3 lbs	Lean boneless lamb
3	Meaty lamb bones

Marinade made from:

Quantity	**Ingredient**
4 tablespoons	Light vegetable oil
$\frac{1}{4}$ c	Cider vinegar
3 tablespoons	Tamarind pulp
to taste	Salt

Puree made from:

Quantity	**Ingredient**
2 tablespoon	Vegetable oil
1 large	White onion
6	Garlic cloves
2 tablespoons	Fresh ginger root, chopped

$\frac{1}{2}$ c	Vegetable oil
3 c	Onion, thinly sliced
1 teaspoon	Ground cumin
1 teaspoon	Ground mustard
3 teaspoons	Turmeric
1 $\frac{1}{2}$ teaspoons	Red pepper
3 teaspoons	Paprika
2 $\frac{1}{2}$ c	Hot water

Method

1. Cut lamb into $\frac{3}{4}$" cubes.
2. Place lamb and the bones in a non-metallic bowl with the four tablespoons of oil, the vinegar, tamarind pulp, and salt. Let it marinate at room temperature for eight hours or, refrigerated, for 24 hours.
3. Put two tablespoons of oil, the onion, garlic, and ginger in an electric blender or food processor and run the machine until a fine pasty puree is formed.
4. Heat the one-half cup of vegetable oil in a large enamel coated skillet over medium-high heat. Add the onions and saute until they are caramel brown, stirring constantly to prevent burning.
5. Add the puree. Reduce the heat and add ground cumin, ground mustard, turmeric, red pepper, and paprika. When the spices begin to sizzle and turn dark, in about 15 seconds, add the lamb and bones. Cook until slightly seared (about ten minutes).
6. Add the water and bring to a boil, then lower the heat and simmer, partially covered, until the meat is very tender (about thirty minutes).
7. Pick out and discard bones.
8. Serve over rice.

11.2 Egg cooked with Meat and Fried (Nargisi Kofta)

Meat:

Quantity	**Ingredient**
1 lb.	Ground lean meat
$\frac{1}{4}$ c	Chopped onion
4 cloves	Chopped garlic
1" piece	Ginger, chopped
$\frac{1}{2}$ t	Turmeric
$\frac{3}{4}$ c	Water
to taste	Salt and pepper

To mix with meat:

Quantity	**Ingredient**
4 T	Besan (chick-pea flour)
1 T	Yogurt
6	Hard boiled eggs
1	Egg for mixing and coating
$\frac{1}{2}$ t	Garam Masala
	Oil for frying

For curry (Masala):

Quantity	**Ingredient**
	Oil or ghee
2	Chopped onions
8	Cloves chopped garlic
2	Tomatoes or equivalent paste
1" piece	Ginger, chopped
$\frac{1}{4}$ c	Yogurt
$\frac{1}{4}$ t	Turmeric
	Green onion
$\frac{1}{2}$ t	Garam Masala
10-15 leaves	Coriander
to taste	Salt and pepper

Method

1. Heat the water and add the meat, onions, ginger, garlic, salt and pepper. Pressure cook for 10 minutes at 15 psi (or 25 min over low heat.

Reduce pressure and drain half the liquid. Add the besan (or $\frac{1}{2}$ c soaked lentils) and cook for 10 minutes. Knead or grind until slightly sticky, mix in egg yolk, Garam Masala and yogurt and knead well.

2. Coat the hard boiled eggs with the above and deep fry.

3. Heat ghee, fry the onions to a golden brown, add garlic, ginger, tomatoes and yogurt and fry well until the Masala is a paste. Add water to the mix if necessary. Add the green sprigs of onion, $1\frac{1}{2}$ c water and cook for 10 minutes covered.

4. When curry is ready, pour into a serving dish, cut the koftas in half and arrange over the curry. Cover and bake at 250 $F°$ for 15-20 minutes.

5. Serve garnished with coriander leaves and Garam Masala.

11.3 Pork Curry

Serves 6 or 8

Quantity	**Ingredient**
1 $\frac{1}{2}$ lb.	Pork
3	Medium onions
2" piece	Ginger
4 cloves	Garlic
2 medium	Tomatoes
2 T	Vinegar
2 t	Salt
$\frac{1}{2}$ t	Garam Masala
2 T	Vindaloo paste (hot)
1 medium	Potatoes
2 c	Water

Method

1. Clean, wash, trim and dry pork. Cut into 1" cubes.

2. Make Masala with onions, ginger, and tomatoes as in chicken curry, etc.

3. Add the vinegar and Vindaloo paste and cook for 2 minutes.

4. Add the pork and pressure cook for 20 minutes, or in a heavy pot for $1\frac{1}{2}$ hours, until the pieces are tender.

5. Cube potatoes, add and cook the potato pieces coated in the liquid.

6. Boil down the amount of water (30 minutes) while the potatoes cook.

11.4 Shahi Korma (Mutton Curry)

Quantity	Ingredient
$1\frac{1}{2}$ lb.	Goat mutton
3	Medium onions
$\frac{3}{4}$ c	Yogurt
4 cloves	Garlic
pinch	Saffron
2 t	Salt
$\frac{3}{4}$ c	Cream
1 oz.	Almonds
$\frac{1}{2}$ c	Oil
1 oz.	Coriander seed
1 t	Red pepper (optional)
$\frac{1}{2}$ t	Garam Masala

Method

1. Clean, wash and dry mutton.

2. Blend coriander seeds, 1 onion, almonds and garlic.

3. Marinade the mutton in above mixture for 2 hrs.

4. Heat oil and fry the remaining thinly sliced onion. Keep aside.

5. Add the mutton and fry until the liquid dries up.

6. Add $\frac{3}{4}$ c hot water and simmer until the meat is almost done ($\frac{3}{4}$ cooked) OR pressure cook at 15 psi for 20 minutes. Reduce pressure. Add salt and pepper.

7. Uncover and dry the liquid.

8. Add beaten yogurt and fry until it leaves oil.
9. Add fried ground onion.
10. Beat the cream. Add soaked or ground saffron.
11. Mix it with the cooked mutton.
12. Add Garam Masala and bake at 250 F° for $\frac{1}{2}$ hour
13. Serve garnished with chopped coriander leaves.

Chapter 12

Desserts and Other Goodies

12.1 Kheer (Vermicelli Pudding)

Recipe from Dalbir Chadda: This has been my all time favorite dessert. Ever since I was very little, I can remember asking for seconds and thirds. What makes this dessert unusual is that it is not as sweet as most Indian desserts. It is fairly simple to make. Make sure that the vermicelli is very fine (angel hair pasta is ok but the very fine vermicelli that can be bought at chinese stores is the best).

Quantity	**Ingredient**
1 stick	Butter
2 handfuls	Very fine vermicelli
4 cups	Milk
1 pint	Whipping cream
1 handful	Raisins
3 tablespoons	Sugar
4	Almonds (optional) peeled and thinly sliced

Method

1. Melt butter in a 4 qt. pot.
2. Break vermicelli into 3" pieces. Over low heat stir vermicelli into butter until it turns light brown.
3. Pour in the milk and stir over medium heat until it boils.

4. Put in the raisins, almonds and sugar.

5. Continue to cook under low heat for 10 minutes.

6. Add whipping cream and continue to cook for a couple of minutes.

7. Remove from heat and, when cool, chill in the refrigerator before serving

12.2 Rice Flour Pudding

6 servings

Quantity	**Ingredient**
4 $\frac{1}{2}$ c	Milk
$\frac{3}{4}$ c	Sugar
2 oz.	Rice flour
6-8 drops	Rose water
1 oz.	Almonds
$\frac{1}{2}$ oz.	Pistachio nuts

Method

1. Blanch (optional) and shred nuts.

2. Mix rice flour into the milk and mix until smooth.

3. Cook over medium heat until a creamy consistency is achieved (20-30 minutes?).

4. Simmer and add sugar and stir for 2-3 minutes more.

5. Cool (in refrigerator for 30 minute) add the rose water, almonds and pistachios (maybe before it cools).

6. Pour into individual dishes and serve.

12.3 Besan Burfi

Quantity	Ingredient
1 c	Besan
1 c	Shortening
1 c	Sugar
4 seeds	Cardamom
	Nuts (optional)

Method

1. Melt shortening in a pan.
2. Turn down heat and add cardamom and Besan.
3. Fry, stirring constantly to prevent burning until it has changed to a brown color and smells done. (Test: a few drops of water sprinkled on it sputters instantly).
4. Turn off the heat and stir in the sugar.
5. Spread $\frac{1}{2}$" thick onto a platter.
6. Cut into diamond shapes after it has cooled down.

12.4 Kheer

Quantity	Ingredient
$\frac{1}{2}$ c	Rice
4 c	Milk
$\frac{1}{4}$ c	Raisins
$\frac{3}{4}$-1 c	Sugar
1 t	Cardamom seeds
$\frac{1}{4}$ c	Shredded blanched almonds
6-8 drops	Rose water
$\frac{1}{2}$ c	Water

Method

1. Wash and drain the rice.

2. Soak in $\frac{1}{2}$ c water for $\frac{1}{2}$ hour.

3. Boil the rice in the same water until it is coated and the water dries up.

4. Add the milk and simmer on low heat for 1 $\frac{1}{2}$ hours.

5. Scrape the sides and bottom frequently to prevent sticking and mash rice while stirring.

6. When it is creamy, add sugar and stir in well.

7. Remove from heat and add crushed cardamom seeds, rose water and shredded almonds.

8. Serve hot or cold decorated with silver leaves (optional). [Silver leaves are VERY FINE, tasteless sheets of silver.]

12.5 Gulab Jamuns (Easy Method)

Quantity	Ingredient
1 c	Bisquick
2 c	Carnation powder
2 c	Water
1 $\frac{1}{2}$ c	Sugar
4 pods	Cardamom
few drops	Rose water
$\frac{1}{2}$ stick	Butter (4 T)
$\frac{1}{8}$ c	Yogurt
	Milk
	Oil for frying

Method

1. Heat butter and pour in a bowl.

2. Add Bisquick, carnation powder and yogurt and blend together.

3. Knead well adding milk if necessary.

4. Make a smooth ball, cover and let rest (30 minutes?).

5. Make 12-14 small balls.

6. Heat the water, add sugar, bring to boil, add cardamom seeds and simmer.

7. Boil, then simmer to reduce the water by half.

8. Heat the oil until hot and fry the balls to a golden brown or until they are dark brown—almost black.

9. Soak in sugar syrup until they double in size (1 hour or overnight)

10. serve hot or cold.

12.6 Suji Halva (Semolina Halva)

4 - 6 servings

Quantity	Ingredient
$\frac{1}{2}$ c	Suji (semolina)
$\frac{1}{2}$ c	Sugar
$\frac{1}{2}$ c	Ghee
1 $\frac{1}{2}$ c	Water
1 oz.	Sliced almonds
1 oz.	Raisins
8	Green cardamoms

Method

1. Boil sugar and water together for 5 minutes.

2. Heat ghee add suji and stir on low heat until mixture becomes light creamy in color and ghee leaves the side of the pan.

3. Add the syrup and stir briskly until it is absorbed in the semolina.

4. Mix in crushed cardamom seeds, almonds, and raisins.

5. Serve hot.

12.7 Sewian (Vermicelli)

Quantity	Ingredient
2 c	Sewian (vermicelli)
$3\frac{1}{2}$ c	Milk
$\frac{3}{4}$ c	Sugar
$\frac{1}{4}$ t	Rose water (or 6-8 small cardamom seeds)
	Ghee

Method

1. Fry the sewian in hot oil until golden brown.
2. Heat the milk to boiling and add the sewian. Cook until the milk is reduced by half.
3. Add sugar and cook on low heat until creamy (about 25 minutes).
4. Remove from the heat. Add in rose water.
5. Decorate with blanched finely shredded almonds and pistachio nuts and silver leaves if desired.

12.8 Carrot Halva

Quantity	Ingredient
4 lbs.	Carrots
$\frac{1}{2}$ gal	Milk
2 c	Sugar
2 c	Carnation milk powder
1 c	Oil
to taste	Nuts

Method

1. Clean and grate the carrots.
2. Heat milk to boiling and add the carrots.

3. Cook until liquid is almost gone, stirring to prevent sticking and burning (3 to 4 hours).

4. Add oil and cook more, stirring often, to roast the carrots well (about $\frac{1}{2}$ hour).

5. Add the powdered milk and sugar and cook until all the liquid is gone and the mass does not stick to the sides.

6. Add the nuts and raisins and turn off the heat.

7. Pour in a serving dish and serve warm or cold. Will keep in the refrigerator for up to 1 week.

12.9 Rasgoola

Quantity	Ingredient
1 L	Homogenized Milk
2 tsp	White Vinegar
$1\frac{1}{2}$ C	Sugar
3 C	Water

Method

1. Bring the milk to a boil and add vinegar to the boiling milk to separate the whey.

2. Throw away the liquid part by sifting the stuff onto a muslin cloth.

3. Pour some cold water over the curd to cool and wash it. Discard the water and hang the cloth for 15-20 minutes to let the excess water drip off.

4. Put the curd in a food processor or blender and blend at high speed to get a smooth consistency. You may add just a little (1 tsp or so) water while blending, if the curd is too dry and will not blend. Be very careful so as not to add any extra water.

5. Remove the paste and make small balls (1-2" in diameter).

6. Boil water in a wide vessel. Make sure that there is at least 2-3" of water in the vessel. If not, add more water and increase the quantity of sugar proportionately. Add sugar to the boiling water to make a light syrup.

7. Continue boiling the syrup and gently drop the curd balls in the boiling syrup. Cook the balls in the boiling syrup for 30-40 minutes.

8. Remove from the heat and let the stuff cool down. Put the balls and the syrup in a storage container and refrigerate (don't freeze).

9. Serve cold.

12.10 Mango Ice Cream

This is a great desert which can be made with very little effort. You can replace the Mango pulp with any other pureed fruit.

Quantity	Ingredient
1 can	Condensed Milk
12 oz.	Whipped cream(Cool whip)
1 can	Mango pulp (Alphonso)

It is very confusing to describe quantities as 1 can. Well, I do not remember the exact numbers so let me describe the sizes. The Mango pulp can is about 6" high and 3" in diameter.I think it is the only size available in an Indian store. The condensed milk can is about 3" high and about 2.5 " in diameter and should be available in your neighbourhood grocery store.

Method

1. Mix all of the pulp, condensed milk and whipped cream in a bowl.

2. Put in the freezer for about 8 hours.

CPSIA information can be obtained
at www.ICGtesting.com
Printed in the USA
LVHW010402290423
745610LV00007B/149